# WELCOME WELL

By Elliot Schulz

# CONTENTS

# WAIVER INFO

The following information contained in this work is for educational and entertainment purposes only and, in no way, is it intended to replace proper medical care. If you have serious condition or an emergency, please seek proper medical treatment as needed. The information provided in this work has been fact-checked and researched to the best ability of the author. Exceptional care was taken to include, edit, and maintain accurate and research-based information while developing this literary work. The author claims no responsibility for each item, action, and topic in this work including but not limited to any omissions, errors, or mistakes that were not intended. In addition, the reader assumes all responsibility participating in any event, practice, or topic discussed in this work. The reader also takes responsibility of any actions taken as a result of reading this book and waives all responsibility from the author legally, medically, or otherwise. Many of the areas discussed in this book are open for interpretation and, thus, different resources may have slightly differing information. The following is what worked best for me, but everyone is different. I have tried, used, and adapted methods from many sources. Be true to yourself and follow your inner guidance.

# INTRODUCTION

Wellness is a large-scale, all-encompassing, almost over-whelming term, ideology, and practice that most, if not all, strive to achieve. How are some people just so breezy with things that come up in their life, while others struggle to get just a small piece of the proverbial "pie"? There are many pieces of the puzzle to look at in regards to wellness that can impact not only health, but your entire life and the life of those around you. Taking into consideration as many pieces of that puzzle of wellness and incorporating as many things as you are able, are comfortable with, and that you deem important can help you achieve your over-all wellness goals as well as escalate your life to that next level you have always been striving for. Let's look into the well of wellness together!

Having a background and experience in modern science and medicine, I have grown up around healthcare but always felt there was more to wellness than just what comes from treatment of ailments from a medical facility. I started getting more involved with learning about things like feng shui, meditation, chakras, and healing crystals. While researching these areas and trying new methods I uncovered, I was fascinated with what developed through applying some practices in my own life and our home.

The vast sources of information on some of these topics can be overwhelming so I have included an appendix of some favorite gurus, books, websites, and resources to help guide you and continue your journey on the road of life.

View these topics as an introductory basis for learning

some of the fundamentals in areas that I have been interested in and wanted to share the information with you. The knowledge I have gained and the teachings I have been so fortunate to receive have changed my life in so many wonderful ways! I can't wait to share that with you!

Visit www.oneboolane.com for a free gift and further information on the topics discussed in this book. Please share your valuable feedback after reading and let me know if you would like more information on specific topics in the feedback section. I appreciate you being here!

# CHAPTER 1 - EDUCATION/ MOTIVATION

You can find out so much about yourself (and the world!) by picking up a book, starting an audiobook, or signing up for a course on a topic you have always been interested in. Make it easy on yourself when getting started ang go with something that you have wanted to know more about. You will be surprised at what emerges once you "crack the surface" on learning. Very often, you may begin to research a certain topic and that may lead you into other areas of interest and this may be the perfect snowball effect to get you into the groove of advancing your skillsets. Keep on reading books, taking courses, and getting degrees and accreditations. You will never regret acquiring more information and knowledge. Tap into the well of wellness!

Personally, I am a big advocate for audiobooks. I find them versatile when being on the go, on a daily commute while you are driving, or getting to and from daily activities. During the time of developing this book, Covid 19 coronavirus has been making some of the daily "normals" suddenly not so normal anymore. But this time that we are in is as good a time as any to start to look more in-depth into the topics in this book.

There are many ways to start on books that don't require any extra money. If you are a smartphone user or have a tablet, many public library systems have access on apps like Libby or

Overdrive where you can borrow books just on your own personal device without having to even go to the library. Audible on Amazon is a great one and has an amazing collection of audiobooks, but there is a monthly fee after your first free credit from them.

Loyal Books offer another collection of audiobooks and features a public domain free content. When all else fails, Google it! You can get connected with some amazing information just through Google, You Tube, and other platforms, but be sure to look at where the content is coming from and maybe check out reviews if you aren't sure of the source(s).

What's that you say? You don't have the time for it? That is all a state of mind – you do have the time for it! Don't make excuses! Making a moment for this will maximize your time in other areas of your life and make everything more meaningful and valuable. Don't make excuses! Everyone has been there with making excuses for things or procrastinating with something over the course of their lives. Some are better with it than others, but the more you are able to curtail putting things off, the better! With everything! If you are debating on doing something, the worst decision you can make is not deciding! The old saying is true, don't put off to tomorrow what you can do today.

Regardless if it is something good, or something that you are dragging your feet on because you don't really want to but know that you have to, you will feel much better to just get it completed and out of the way. You are here reading this because you are wanting to focus on yourself, your health, family, life's journey, or whatever the case is. It is important to just take the time and do what you have been meaning to do. Have you been thinking of starting something but weren't sure if it was right? Just go ahead and get it started! You can always decide once you have the project going if it is something that will turn out the way you intended or perhaps it will be something that will change your mind. You will never know unless you try.

# CHAPTER 1 RECAP: THINGS TO PONDER AND PRACTICE

1. Spare a moment of your day and research a topic you are interested in.
2. Decide if you would like to start a book or course on the topic.
3. Don't put off doing what you have been meaning to start.
4. Travel your own journey into higher learning, wellness, and harmony.
5. It is all about the journey and not the destination!

# CHAPTER 2 - INSTINCT

Your own instinct can save your life! If you are feeling a certain way in the pit of your stomach, that is probably your 3rd eye or intuition telling you about that decision. Go with your gut instincts! Have you ever answered a question and had a feeling what the answer was, but then you over-thought the question, sat on it too long, let your mind wander with it, only to select the wrong answer in the end?! Moral of the story: trust your "gut" (aka intuitive senses).

Our 3rd eye or intuition is something that each of us have within; however, over the course of centuries of science and education, it is repressed. Therefore, it is something that needs to be exercised and acknowledged to function properly again. The more you use your intuition and focus on developing it, the better it will become. Luckily, there are some straightforward ways to help get it activated again and to initialize the processes of using it on a more regular basis.

One of my favorite ways to help to activate the third-eye intuition is to observe the sunrise and sunset. I am not saying to stare directly into the sun; please don't! That could lead to injury to the eye or worse, but just to take in the beauty of the serene sunrise or sunset has an effect on the intuition senses and third eye.

This sense may be related to the pineal gland. Science and research show that this gland produces hormones for the body; however, its full functionality can be sometimes rather mystic. Although the third eye is said to be located between your eyes, above the bridge of your nose, the pineal gland is actually more in the middle of your brain technically. More new age research suggests they are perhaps somehow related.

Another way to boost the intuitive sense is simply by being around the colors purple and dark blue. These colors are indicative of the third-eye chakra as well as the crown chakra colors. To improve upon your intuition, simply wear, have, and use the color in your day-to-day life with the intention on boosting your third-eye senses. Put a purple item on your desk, wear a purple shirt, pick up some purple jewelry, etc.

You can also take a moment to close your eyes and picture the color dark blue in between your eyes as a sort of radar or antenna that is assisting in your navigation of life. By doing so, you are actually doing a mini meditation on your chakra.

I have also found that putting something purple by your nightstand at night can help you to remember your dreams, and again, it's possible it is all related to the third eye and intuition. Dark blue or purple hued crystals and natural minerals are wonderful ways to assist your third-eye chakra to its full potential. Such examples include but are not limited to iolite, amethyst, blue sodalite, and lapis lazuli to name a few. Use, wear, and/or carry with you those types of crystals to help enhance and activate the powers within your third eye. What matters most is putting your intention in a focused manner to boost that sense, regardless on which method you choose. More on meditation, crystals, and chakras to come.

# CHAPTER 2 RECAP: THINGS TO PONDER AND PRACTICE

1. Everyone has an intuitive sense it just needs activation and regular usage.
2. Listen to your gut instinct and focus on that for development of your intuition.
3. Take in sunrise, sunsets, and nature.
4. Wear or use the color purple or dark blue in your daily life *with intention.*
5. Close your eyes and picture the area in between your eyes as a dark blue or purple-colored radar taking in pertinent information (meditation with your third eye).

# CHAPTER 3 - CHAKRAS

If you are not familiar with the chakras of the body, you may be questioning the last chapter that focused on the third-eye chakra. I started with that point as many are familiar with that term even if they aren't exactly sure on chakras. Chakra (pronounced either Shock-Rah or Chock-Rah) refers to the 7 sections or wheels of the body. These are the governing energy centers that help regulate and facilitate wellness throughout the body. They work both together and separately and are thought of as wheels that are constantly in motion.

Just like well-oiled machines with wheels and gears, chakras work best when they are thought-after and cared for appropriately. Your body, mind, and spirit also are in that same boat as these all work best when well-taken-care of. Each of the seven chakras represent a different part of the body and have different names, colors, and ways you can enhance that aspect of your own chakra system. There are entire books, courses, and accreditations on chakras, but I will give you a basis of the concepts and some ways to work on them. However, you should note, this is a just scratches the surface of a very in-depth topic.

Let's start from the bottom to the top. The lower most base chakra is called the root chakra and is located at the base of the spine. When thinking of chakras, it is important to start at this base point as the chakras can be looked at as somewhat of a hierarchy of needs. The root chakra is represented with the red, black, and even brown tones. This chakra has to do with grounding and being in a place of feeling safe, having nourishment (food), and security. Security could be interpreted as having money or the ability to make and do transactions that benefit you, but should not be regarded in *only* that particular way. Money does not necessarily buy happiness nor does money necessarily buy a balanced and grounded root chakra either.

Working on your root chakra can be as easy as being more mindful of the way you are feeling in regards to health and safety. It is linked to your ability to have a means of feeling safe (environment, safe home, etc.). To boost this chakra, you can incorporate the colors listed above into your wardrobe, jewelry, nail polish, or personal space. You can also work on your root chakra by spending time outdoors, eating nourishing foods, and being extra mindful of your body's needs. Do a mini-meditation by closing your eyes and picturing feet being connected to the earth with roots that ground you to mother nature. Even a few moments of closing your eyes and doing this visualization can help you to be more grounded.

Next chakra is the sacral chakra and is located in the area near the belly button. This wheel of energy is represented with tones of the color orange and is connected to our inner passion, energy, and vitality both on physical and mental/emotional levels. You can strengthen this chakra by working on creative projects that use your natural artistic abilities that are part of you! Do you have something you have been thinking of creating but haven't started on (remember that from the first chapter on motivation)? Get out there and begin using your creativity, this is a wonderful boost for your sacral chakra. Also, as always, wearing the color orange in clothing, jewelry, and using/carrying/wearing orange-colored crystals or minerals.

Above sacral chakra, next up is the solar plexus chakra. The solar plexus chakra is located about halfway between the heart and the belly button. This chakra is represented with the color yellow and has to do with our confidence and power levels. Have you heard of working your "core" for exercise? The solar plexus is your essential "core" of power, so exercising and focusing on that area is a wonderful way of boosting that area. Aside from wearing the color of the chakra, healthy foods that match the color chakra you are wanting to strengthen also work wonders to boost that area. Focus on your inner core during a meditation and picture the yellow wheel spinning and being strong! More on meditation in a later chapter, but all chakras can be strengthened with meditation.

The heart chakra is the next above the solar plexus. This chakra is represented with the color green and can act as an aligner for all the chakras of the body. This deeply meaningful and literally "heart felt" chakra is, not surprisingly, strengthened with love, compassion, and the ability to be empathetic. You can "feel" for a person and be compassionate while still protecting yourself from getting into a lower vibration (i.e., taking on that person's pain or experiences of sorrow). By caring, you are making your heart chakra stronger and more rooted.

Selflessly giving to others is also a wonderful way to boost the heart chakra. Wearing green, eating healthy greens, and using crystals that are green, pink, or have a combination of the aforementioned colors are also wonderful ways to work on that area as well. Hold your hand over your heart and meditate for a moment, feel your heart beat, appreciate the wonder of your human body to have this marvelous organ that works all by itself without any thought. Go one step further, be thankful of all your organs and your body as a whole for getting you through each day and to this very moment in time. You are in the exact place you are to be right now.

Next is the throat chakra. The 5$^{th}$ chakra is an especially important area (actually they are all important) but this one deals with communications and our ability to verbalize what we need to, when we need to. It is the meeting place of our inner voice and our vocalizing abilities. Frog in your throat? You may have a somewhat blocked throat chakra. It is represented by the color light blue, and can also deal with the back of your neck area where many of us carry the burden of stress or anxiousness.

Within this chakra area is the mouth. This is a good reminder to take care of your teeth! Oral hygiene is important for overall well-being but this is emphasized when taking a look at the throat chakra. Floss and brush frequently, and don't forget to brush your tongue! Schedule that dentist appointment you have been putting off! Strengthen your smile and, at the same time, your throat chakra.

Working with, wearing, and using light-blue-colored crystals or minerals (jewelry, touch stones, or tumbled stones in your pocket) is another way of working on the throat chakra. Crystal expert Heather Askinosie of the book *Crystal Muse* and website www.energymuse.com, uses a wonderful practice of taking a piece of selenite (a natural mineral) and waving that around the different chakra area(s) that she is working on. Taking that selenite and moving it around the outside of your throat area is a method of clearing your throat chakra (and help to clear that frog from your throat). I love this practice with all chakra areas and find the clearing method works well when you picture energetically clearing away blockages and grounding them back to mother earth.

Onto the third-eye chakra (technically the 6$^{th}$ chakra), which was previously discussed in the intuition chapter. This is another especially important one. Yes, yes, they are all important! This is your instinct or your "gut feeling" that you get or may have felt a twinge of in the past but ignored. Don't ignore your gut instinct! That instinct was given to every one of us and is a part of everyone.

Historically it was utilized in past civilizations as survival instinct on a day-to-day basis. Think of cave-man-times when just making it through each day would require quite a lot of advanced thinking and survival instinct. Obviously, they did not have cell phones giving directions or telling if a certain plant is poisonous or bringing up the weather if there is going to be a big, dangerous storm coming!

Over the ages, our technological advancements have helped humankind develop further in many ways and have brought us so many useful tools (like those cell phones). However, the utilization of our third-eye sense has been downplayed over centuries by education and science. One way to reconnect would be to do a mini meditation and focus on the area in between your eyes; picture a dark blue/purple wheel turning. Get comfortable either sitting or lying back, and focus on your breath. Breathe normally, but try quieting thoughts other than the thought of the third-eye area. Picture it as a turning wheel that is like a radar, helping to navigate your path.

As mentioned with the other chakras, you can wear the color dark blue and purple and work with this charka. The third-eye chakra color is technically "indigo" so any deep, dark, blue, or violet crystals like those mentioned in the chapter on intuition will help your intuition sense. Even lightly tapping on that area in between your eyes can help awaken that sense, and as mentioned earlier, taking in the sunrise and sunset can strengthen this area as well.

Finally, the seventh chakra (or crown chakra) is at the top of your head and also has been known to be associated with the pineal gland, as was previously mentioned about the third-eye chakra. These two top-of-the-body chakras also share some similar color representations as the crown is associated with light violet and purple colors but also is additionally associated with white. Picture the crown as the center of being peaceful and feeling a connection to the spiritual realm as well as one's divine inner self. Being at peace, being thankful, and being balanced are feelings associated with having a smooth functioning crown chakra. Taking a moment of silence and doing a meditation, even for a minute (or longer is best) and focusing on this chakra is a way to improve it. A great visualizing practice is to picture a white light coming down from the sun, stars, and/or moon and filling your body with pure light.

This should be the last chakra to focus on as you should

work on tending to lower chakras and balancing and aligning the lower levels first. Just like building a house, you wouldn't start with the roof! Same is true for chakras and a solid foundation to build upon is the place to start. This information on chakras is by no means all-encompassing of the information out there but it is a solid start on the path of knowledge. You can research the chakras and find more information about the history, the Sanskrit symbols that represent each, as well as other activities you could work on if you find an area that you would like to touch up on. If you feel drawn towards a certain color, design, flower, crystal, piece of jewelry, etc., it could be that particular associated chakra in your body calling out for a little boost! Listen to your instinct.

# CHAPTER 3 RECAP: THINGS TO PONDER AND PRACTICE

*Your chakras are wheels in motion that govern various parts of the body*

1. Root chakra (number 1 chakra) located at base of spine, health related, tied to basic needs and necessities.
   i. Focus on wearing the colors red, black, brown (earth) tones, eating healthy foods, and meditating picturing your feet "grounding" into the earth.
2. Sacral chakra (number 2 chakra) is located near the belly button, depicted with the color orange, represents your passion, energy, and creativity.
   i. Focus on doing creative tasks and projects, also being conscious of wearing or using the color orange in your daily activities.
3. Solar plexus chakra (number 3 chakra) is halfway between belly button and heart, is the color yellow, represents power and confidence.
   i. Focus on eating foods of that color, exercising (specifically on the "core"), wearing the color yellow, and meditating picturing the yellow core of your body being strong and sturdy.

4. Heart chakra (number 4 chakra) is depicted with the colors green or pink and represents love, compassion, and your hearts desires.

     i. Focus on being selfless with those around you, being giving, and treating others with respect and compassion. Also being grateful for every little thing in your life and also affirming with meditation focusing on your heart and body.

5. Throat chakra (number 5 chakra) includes your throat, neck, and mouth area.

     i. Focus on incorporating the color light blue into your wardrobe, being thankful for your smile and your voice, and also being diligent with oral hygiene. As with any of the chakras you can do a meditation focusing on that area.

6. Third eye chakra (number 6 chakra) is the area in between the eyes and is the intuition central of the body.

     i. Focus on using the color dark blue and/or violet in your wardrobe and day-to-day life. Also trust your inner instinct and remain attuned to what your body tells you and meditate while focusing on that area.

7. Crown chakra (number 7 chakra) top of the head chakra that is represented with the colors white and purple/violet and is the spirituality side of one's true self.

     i. Focus on being thankful, work on including the color purple or white into your life, and meditate with particular intent on picturing pure white healing, energizing light going to and from the top of your head (beaming to and from the universe through the head and body).

# CHAPTER 4 – MEDITATION & PRAYER

Meditation is the practice of taking a duration of time to be quiet and still and to focus on working to slow the mind. The last chapter introduced doing some meditation practices to boost certain aspects of your chakras and your entire chakra system in general. Our day-to-day grind is surely a busy one! From daily tasks like hustling to and from work, doing work around the house, taking care of loved ones, children, family, pets, there are a lot of responsibilities that each of us take on. It is little wonder why the feelings of anxiety and being overwhelmed come up. For many, we are at maximum capacity. This is why taking the time to meditate is even more important.

In order to be our best for others, we must first focus on ourself and being the best for us. My mind is always trying to be on a million things at once. Granted this can be very productive in getting things accomplished and checked off the daily to-do's; however, this practice is not exactly always helpful and is certainly not a practice of being mindful. I know it seems counterintuitive if you are already pressed for time to "make time" for a practice of mediating, but this self-care practice is particularly important. Even if there is just a minute or two's worth of time, close your eyes and focus on your breath. Just a minute is all it takes to start to make a difference. I have found a multitude of benefits from meditation including increased focus and awareness, decreased blood pressure, increased sense of stability, increased patience, and the list goes on. Start with a minute or a few minutes and gradually work your way up to longer durations of time.

Once again, there are many different resources out there to guide you to a meditation practice that you like. There is a plethora of videos on YouTube that feature guided meditations as well as videos featuring diverse types of relaxing music, spa music, or megahertz music. Specific megahertz frequencies have effects on various parts of the brain and can help to get you to a relaxed state of mind. Maybe something that features someone telling you how or when to breathe helps you, or maybe just something with a soft soothing nature sound is right for you.

Go with what works, and what feels best for you. Your body will adjust to being able to be quiet for a time and with your mind focusing on your breath, you will slowly be able to let the busy thoughts float away. If you happen to start thinking of something during your time mediating, that is ok! Don't fret about it, just acknowledge the thought and refocus on your breathing. If it helps, you can count: breathe in for 4 seconds, hold for 4 seconds, and breathe out for 4 seconds. And repeat.

Another visualization method is to focus on picturing the air being a purifying white cloud, similar to how your breath would look like on a chilly winters' day. Picture positive, peaceful, pure white air coming into your body and breathe in through your nose, and out through your mouth. As you exhale out through your mouth, let any negativity, anxious, or unhealthy energy leave your body. Work on this for at least 10 breaths and feel your body relax and anxiousness start to ease.

While meditation might be something new that you are starting to explore; there is a term that may resonate more with you, prayer. Regardless of your personal spiritual beliefs, prayer can be part of a meditation or can be considered a form of meditation by itself. Prayer is a powerful practice that anyone can utilize in addition to or in conjunction with meditation. It involves some of the same techniques to quiet the mind while keeping thoughts on reflectivity, thankfulness, and/or focusing on others and directing health and healing energy.

Everything in the universe is comprised of energy and it really does make an impact to send your warm thoughts and vibrations to those in need. Whether it is in the form of a prayer or meditation, whatever you choose to call it is up to you. Helping others is an experience that adds enrichment to your life. In helping others, you are unintentionally fueling your own manifestations.

# CHAPTER 4 RECAP: THINGS TO PONDER AND PRACTICE

1. Meditation is beneficial for mind, body, and spirit.
2. Start with trying one or two minutes and work your way up to 10-15+ mins.
3. Begin with focusing on breath; breathing in positive light and energy.
4. If thoughts stray, acknowledge them, and move back to focus on breathing.
5. Try adding specific meditation music to help get in the zone.
6. Pair meditation and prayer together while your mind is clear and free.

# CHAPTER 5 - MINDFULNESS

Being mindful is another wellness strategy you may have heard but may not exactly know what it is or what it represents. Mindfulness is to focus mental activity on one task at hand, and to enjoy the present moment. What are you doing right now? Reading or listening to this book, yes, but is your mind also going 100 other places and drifting off to think of your to-do list, picking up groceries, what is for supper, taking out the dog, etc.? Multi-tasking and mindfulness are on exact opposite ends of the spectrum.

To be mindful is to enjoy and appreciate the thing you are doing and working on in the exact moment. This can be done by taking the time to sort your thoughts, slow down, and enjoy your current activity, whatever it may be. Doing so will really make a wonderful impact on your entire day. Start with that one thing you are doing at the moment and then try to remember being mindful throughout your day. Watch what a difference mindfulness makes!

If you are at all like me, even when I'm doing something wonderful like a moment of something special, I am still thinking of what the next activity is on the agenda. I catch myself often and, as I have said earlier, I am always learning and working on re-programming for a greater good. Being mindful is something that takes time to work on and practice. Don't be worried if it is not something you automatically can turn on or off overnight. Just as it has been programmed in for us to be on the go, so too will programming be necessary to be mindful. Take a moment now to realize and appreciate what you are doing before jumping into the next activity.

You can be excited about the other aspects that are coming during your day while still be mindful. The adage about it being about "the little things" applies here; be appreciative of the little things. Moreover, *notice* the little things. If you are rushing from one thing to the next you are likely on a path to missing out on some beautiful moments and messages throughout your day. Appreciate your ability to be doing what you are doing at this very moment. Appreciate the opportunity to be at the very place you are right now, and doing the very activity that you are doing. Appreciate the smells, the sensory values, and being alive and on this amazing earth to enjoy those very things.

Perhaps you are not doing your most favorite thing and are wondering how and why you would appreciate doing that particular thing. Just appreciate that you have that one thing that illustrates and highlights all the other things that you enjoy doing more. This will make you appreciate those all the further.

An easy way to be more mindful consistently is to, again, MEDITATE! A little meditation can go a long way and can help in so many different aspects of everyday life.

# CHAPTER 5 RECAP: THINGS TO PONDER AND PRACTICE

1. Mindfulness is focused appreciation for the present.
2. Take time and enjoy each moment.
3. Be mindful about being mindful – it takes practice.
4. Meditate.

# CHAPTER 6 - ZEN DEN

As you start making meditation part of your daily practice, you may want to set aside a particular part of your home as your designated meditation area. I like to call this space the zen den. This is a sacred space that you dedicate as the area where you meditate. Granted not all meditations necessarily have to be conducted in this area as you may wish to meditate outside when available, or take a moment wherever you are in the day and have a mini meditation. Still, it is helpful to have a space with some serene qualities that assist in getting into the mindful meditation zone.

The best way to begin the process of creating this space is to select the area that you are choosing to make into your meditation zone or zen den. Once that area of the room, or entire room, has been selected, it is time to clean! Start to declutter, organize, and go through the contents of the room. Has it been a while since you went through the items in that area? Time to edit that space and get it to a point of comfort both visually and energetically.

Start with the larger items first like furniture. Move things around to get them to coincide with the vision of your serene space. Then focus on the smaller items and place them in organized areas in or around what fits best with your current rooms, methods, and categories. Next, clean, clean, and clean some more! Dust, vacuum, get rid of spider webs, touch up marks on the walls, wipe down furniture and anything else that energetically can hinder your special space. Starting with the bigger items and moving to the smaller ones follows the most logical decluttering methodology. When you are working on this you are not only making improvements on your selected area for meditation but you are also boosting the feng shui. More on that later in this book.

When you have your area organized and cleaned you can start to add some materials that help make it your special place. You could add soothing pictures or tapestries that take you away to a zone of relaxation. Perhaps burning certain candles or diffusing essential oils will take you to that spa-like place. You can incorporate a little bit of everything. Burning sage, palo santo, incense, and candles can also act as an energetic cleanse in this area as well as setting the mood and tone for your relaxing zen den.

Personally, I have some meditation-inspired tapestries up on the walls with depictions of the different chakras and their corresponding colors and Sanskrit symbols. I also have several selections of crystals and natural minerals represented here and use them as both décor as well as tools for meditation. Put some comfortable furniture around, if you choose, so that you can sit or lay back and enjoy your moments of slowing your racing mind and thoughts.

One of my favorite methods energy clearing is to burn some sage and fan it to the corners of the room with a feather. This is a wonderful way to freshen the air and the energy in any location of the house, car, or virtually any space that could use a lift. During the practice of burning sage, I vent a window to clear out the old energy. I should also note that, when starting, I will run the sage smoke around my body to cleanse myself of any stagnant energy before moving onto the room or space.

Later, or sometimes the next day, I will burn some palo santo (holy wood) to "lock in" the good vibrations and draw in positive energy. I follow the same process with the palo santo step as I do with the sage; using the smoke to first purify myself before moving onto wafting the smoke into the corners of the room to lock in the clean, fresh vibrations. Once you begin to practice using some of these tools you will discover which methods are best for you.

There are sage and palo santo candles, essential oils, and air freshening sprays out there that can and will do the same freshening of your space as the methods above. Candles and essential oils are great tools in space clearing as well as setting the mood in your zen den. Do what works best for you and feels right. Use your intuition.

# CHAPTER 6 RECAP: THINGS TO PONDER AND PRACTICE

1. Select the room or area to establish your zen den.
2. Create a space of serenity and clean, declutter, and organize the space.
3. Add in items like soothing art, crystals, incense, candles, etc.
4. Cleanse yourself and your space with sage/palo santo/or similar incense or herb(s).
5. Enjoy your space! Set time aside to meditate.

# CHAPTER 7 - CRYSTALS

I have been into crystals, rocks, and minerals since I was little. There was a local rock shop downtown in the small town that I grew up in, that I would take my allowance money to purchase tumbled stones and crystals that caught my eye. I even had my very own rock tumbler that I would work with. Over the course of several weeks, which seemed like an eternity back then, I would switch out the different sand (grit) to polish the stones like the ones you see in stores. I had large basins full of them, and unfortunately do not have those originals anymore from when I was a kid, but I do have a vast collection of amazing gems, crystals, and jewelry that I use every day for a variety of purposes. I am continuously acquiring new pieces as they come along, adding them to my growing collection of useful tools to navigate the day.

Crystals are helpful tools in your day-to-day life. They can serve many different purposes from helping during difficult or stressful times to assisting in bringing about energy and vitality. Each stone or crystal has a unique structure, makeup, and a unique vibration. There are literally thousands of different varieties and there are numerous informative books that cover the bases of their makeup more in depth, just like the previous topics. My goal is to introduce them to you so you also can begin using them in areas of your life and bring them into a daily usefulness. Like us, they are happy when they are being of service.

Along with their unique vibrations and energy, each carry certain characteristics that can help us use them in different ways, for different purposes. Again, there is a lot of information out there on each specific crystal type; however, I feel as though a portion of the information available could be left open for interpretation. For example, amethyst is documented to be associated with the crown chakra at the top of your head; however, to me, I feel like it opens up and assists the third-eye chakra. Where one definition may tell you what metaphysical properties the mineral typically represents, you may feel a certain way towards it that differs from what you read. This is totally common and 100% ok! Think of that as your own intuition telling you what your body needs.

If you are drawn to a particular piece for the color, shape, size, etc. – it could be your body calling out for what it could use at that moment. I am frequently very fascinated when selecting a certain mineral that I am drawn to and then later looking up and referencing information on it, only to discover it exactly correlates to something that is going on currently in my life. The crystals know!

When starting out, crystals work best when you follow a couple steps in caring for them. First, anytime you receive a new piece, cleanse it before working with it. There are several different methods for cleansing including putting it on top of the soil of a healthy house plant overnight, simply buffing it with a cloth or rag, or by immersing it in the smoke of burning sage, palo santo, or incense.

Another method of cleansing is submersing it under running water or placing it in a container of salt water for 12-24 hours. However, use the last two methods (involving water) with caution and only after looking up information on that particular piece from a noteworthy source before placing in water/salt water. Not all crystals or minerals can be submerged into salt water and some may even be somewhat water soluble or can corrode if introduced to water or salt water.

The next step, after cleansing, is to decide what you want

the crystal to assist you with. Each crystal has known metaphysical properties that sometimes have dated back centuries from previous civilizations. While most of these characteristics can be found in resources online, via apps, or in books; your own vibration and energy will tell you which crystals to use. Our body's needs and the vibrational energy of crystals form an almost magnetic-like-draw that will show you to the correct crystals to use. Look up pictures from your favorite researching methods and also look at what that crystal's properties are. You can also look up local rock, mineral, and crystal shops that are in your area. A visit to one of these shops would provide you with a further link to the selected stones that you can be working with.

When programming your crystals for your desired usage or intention, it helps to know a bit about them and what their known usages have been as they are all documented as having specific functions already. Just as everybody is different, every crystal is a little different too and can function for multiple purposes depending on the individual. Think of programming or setting intention to them as almost a computer program you are setting on your device.

Modern day-to-day electronics are partially made up of silica, quartz, gold, copper and silver. Many hand-held devices have liquid crystal displays (or LCD as it is commonly referred to) so almost everyone has been using crystals and minerals all along, just in other forms.

Charging the stones is another practice that you should do frequently to keep them in tip top shape, especially if you are using them frequently or, alternatively, have not used them in a long time. Charge them by placing in the window to bask in the sunlight and moonlight or place them on a slab of selenite which is a natural "charging" crystal. You can also place them outside to capture the direct sunlight or moonlight for a few hours but only if you have a safe area to do so to ensure they don't get stolen!

After cleansing and charging in natural light or with selenite, you must then give your crystal tool the definite purpose or intention that you are wanting to program. Hold the crystal in your hand and envision the action you wish to have it assist you with. This could be a large stone, small crystal or geode, or a piece of jewelry that is made from a natural mineral. Envision the outcome you wish to achieve by working with the crystal and every time you see it or touch it, be reminded of what are you planning to accomplish.

Selenite is one crystal that I will mention specifically as it should be in everyone's crystal toolbox. I don't plan on going over each of the thousands of distinct species out there, but this one is a perfect place to begin if you are just getting your game going with these amazing gifts from nature. As stated earlier in the book, use your inner guidance in selecting which pieces are right for you. Did you look up and find that local rock and mineral shop that is in your area? That is an excellent place to start, and likely the associates there would be more than happy to assist in guiding you in your journey to discovering new tools and resources.

While shopping local is always great to support local economies and business owners; you can also begin your searches online with picking out different things that catch your eye. However, this is not always a perfect shopping equation as you are not able to energetically feel the vibration of the crystal in the same way you are when you are at a store viewing, holding, and being drawn to something. That being said, this book was developed during the time of the Covid-19 corona virus and online shopping has become an important way of being able to access things while helping to minimize risks. I have often bought pieces online after viewing them and researching the vendor as well as the specific properties of the piece that I am looking at.

# CHAPTER 7 RECAP: THINGS TO PONDER AND PRACTICE

1. Cleanse crystals before working with them by immersing in smoke, buffing with a cloth, or placing on the soil of a healthy houseplant overnight.
2. Charge crystals often (and after cleansing) in sunlight, moonlight, or on selenite.
3. Crystals that draw your eye are calling for you.
4. Research properties of the crystals and program your intentions accordingly.
5. Program by holding the crystal and saying aloud or in your head your intentions.

# CHAPTER 8 - FENG SHUI

What if someone told you that by moving things around in your home you could become healthier? Or if you were told that by cleaning up some spaces in and around your house that your family could be thriving, your finances flourishing, and each and every area of your life could be in a perfect harmony of success, health, and wealth? Essentially these are some effects of feng shui in a nut shell. I have outlined a few general tips on several of the different popular areas that most tend to focus on with regards to feng shui.

Feng shui translated to English means wind and water, and was adapted from ancient China. The term and practice are essentially referring to the adaptation to creating harmony in your home, and therefore, that harmony translates into your life. There are numerous practices and different interpretations of feng shui that you could spend weeks upon weeks on doing research. Because this was something that has been adapted from an Eastern culture into Western civilization, many of the translations of the methods are somewhat open to interpretation.

If you would like to get more in depth with feng shui, there are dedicated books and courses on each of the specific areas, methods, and practices that they comprise of. I have an online certification in one course that taught the basic principles of feng shui and have read many books on it. And, as stated earlier, I am a life-long-learner and always learning new things. Still, I wanted to give you some of the basic principles so you too can get your feet wet on the topic and begin to use it in your home and experience some amazing magic that it offers.

To start, there are different bagua grids which are maps or layouts of feng shui that you can use as a template over the outline of your home. Typically they are split up into 9 different areas that include wealth and prosperity, fame and reputation, relationships, family, health, creativity, knowledge, career, and finally, travel and helpful people. One is a layout of a square that is broken off into the 9 smaller square areas, and the other popular grid layout is in the shape of an octagon. Both include essentially the same 9 areas so it is just a matter of choice of which grid layout you feel most drawn to using your inner guidance.

Some grids that are available include different titles for the areas of the bagua. I have seen some refer to the area directly to the back of the residence called the "inspiration" area instead of the "fame and reputation" area. But in either case, to find out more on the different spaces of your house you will essentially apply that bagua map as a blueprint over the layout of your home to determine which section of the house applies to that corresponding area of feng shui.

Another important thing to look when getting started is the plumbing in your home. Does everything function properly as it should? Regardless of which area of the bagua map the plumbing fixtures land in, all should be in perfect working order. No leaky faucets, toilets, or drains because, in the world of feng shui, that would represent losses of money or wages. An easy way to remember this translation is picturing the saying "money going down the drain". Fixing these issues may cost some money to repair but eventually you will end up saving money that is lost by the leaky fixtures.

One step further is to tie a piece of red string, tape, or ribbon around the outgoing pipes that lead out of the sink, drain, etc. Red is a stop sign for chi, or energy, and therefore stops the chi (aka money) from wanting to leave. The chi is then redirected as energy and encouraged to recirculate through the home. After learning this technique, I tried it and have been pleased with the positive results. The red ribbon or tie can be out of sight so it doesn't draw attention or look out of place. I used industrial grade red tape (the thicker kind that allows you to cut it easily) and cut small strips big enough to wrap around the out-going plumbing drain and went around the house with them.

Aside from assessing the plumbing, another item that should be looked at when beginning Feng shui is the front door of the house. What does the front door look like on your home? Is the door itself clean, tidy, and functioning properly? How does the walkway or steps leading up to the door look? Clutter, old newspapers, dead foliage, dust, cobwebs in this, or any, area could be affecting yourself and those that dwell within the home. Clean every nook and cranny of the front door area and the front entry way and watch the positive impact it has on your job/career. Don't worry if this all sounds like something that is way out there, trust that it truly does work – just try it and see!

As mentioned, a segment of one of the basic principles with Feng Shui relates to the chi (or energy) flow. This energy into, out of, and throughout your home helps to regulate and facilitate the proper day-to-day functions of your life as well as for those that dwell within the home. Getting back to that cluttered front door area, chi or money, coming into your home (and therefore life) could be held up on the way in if there is debris blocking a clear path into the front door. Similarly, if the door is broken or has a problem functioning, that could block the chi or money coming into the lives of the home dwellers. Again, that front area of where the main door to the house is considered to be the career area, regardless if you primarily use a different door to enter the house.

When looking at or coming in through the front door, the left most rear corner of the house is considered the prosperity and wealth corner. This is a key area to make sure that things are in order if you are looking at increasing your wealth and success. Ensure the area is tidy and clean in this entire space; making sure each corner and hidden area is rid of dust, dirt, and anything that could block the chi from having a harmonious flow. Healthy house plants in this, or any, area of the home can be an excellent way to boost the over-all feng shui factor.

In addition, things that represent prosperity to you would be good additions to this space such as gold and silver colored décor items, pyrite stones, framed art, and anything that represents wealth to you. These items you add should be tasteful and match the décor of the home without cluttering. Clutter is a chi blocker and should be avoided in every area. Items in the color purple can also be added to this area to boost the wealth and success factor as well, but don't over-do it by adding too many things as feng shui is all about having harmony and balance.

The relationship corner of the home is the rear right corner, regardless if this is the area of any bedroom of the house. In our house, the relationship corner is actually our garage. To boost this area and to strengthen your relationship with your spouse, significant other, or to draw in love to your life; you will use some of the same principles that applied in the prosperity corner. Clean this space from top to bottom, even if it is your garage or storage space - clean it as if it is a room of your house! Clean every corner, organize, dust, vacuum, and create a space that is pleasing to your eye. Use your intuition here and go with a style that matches what your own personal tastes are – you are intuitive! You could incorporate some of the colors red, or pink, or tan/beige/natural skin-tones if they are not already represented here.

# CHAPTER 8 RECAP: THINGS TO PONDER AND PRACTICE

1. Feng shui translates to wind and water and focuses on harmony in your home.
2. Use a bagua map as a blueprint to outline each feng shui section of the house.
3. Clean and declutter each area with intention.
4. Check plumbing fixtures for leaks as well as the front door functionality.

# CHAPTER 9 – JOURNALING & LAW OF ATTRACTION

There are numerous benefits to picking up a notepad or dedicated journal and jotting down a few thoughts each day. I have found doing so has similar health benefits to meditation such as increasing mental focus and it could even assist in outlining your exact desired life path and manifestations. Write down specifics of dreams, desires, and wishes and write them as if they are happening or have already happened. This is sometimes called scripting and can leave you feeling refreshed and invigorated. You are scripting your own life and making a list of orders to have the universe fulfill.

Remember looking at a toy catalog as a kid when the Christmas sales begin to come out in the season preceding the holidays? I used to circle the toys that I wanted and would sometimes cut them out so my family would know exactly what I wanted under the tree that year. Think of the universe as your holiday catalog that you are making selections from! What types of things do you desire? What are the feelings that you will have when experiencing those dreams? Work journaling/scripting into your daily activities. Try to do at least 5 to 10 minutes of journaling or fit in small increments during the day as time allows.

Pair journaling with meditation for a powerful means of grounding and becoming self-aware. Make daily practices and you will receive astounding results. Set an intention of writing down things that you are thankful for and also tie in things that you are wanting to bring about in your life and you will start to rewire your subconscious into setting off patters that will begin manifesting your deepest desires. You can work your way up to writing a couple pages per day, or set a timer for writing while making it a daily practice.

For a turbo boost on the path to manifesting, grab a couple of your favorite crystals and give them the intention of helping achieve the desired outcome. Hold them during writing in your non dominant hand or place them nearby so their frequency and vibration can be felt. Remember to set intention to those crystals that you are working with to get the maximum benefit!

Although it is not necessarily magic, I like to believe there is some magic along with putting out to the universe your desired dreams and outcomes. Especially when you are able to get into the vibrational frequency and feel as if it has already happened. Grab onto those feelings of how it *will* be *when* those dreams come to realization. This practice will put your vibration out to the universe so to match that of what you desire. More than just setting up your desires, journaling will allow you to start to make those dreams a reality by opening up pathways for you to be able to take steps to getting to that desired outcome. This is part of what is typically referred to as the Law of Attraction.

The law of attraction was helped to popularity by the docu-film *The Secret* by Rhonda Byrne and while that is a great introduction, the practice is sometimes easier said than done. The takeaway is that you are what you think about. If your thoughts are focused on positive things, your goals, dreams and ambitions; you are drawing those things into your life. If you are grateful for what you have, more will increasingly find its way to you. Gratitude goes a long way.

Being thankful for the things that you have will bring upon more good things. Put your wishes and dreams out there, but do not continuously harp on them. You must be careful to put out to the universe what you wish for and not dwell on the how or why. Dwelling on the how and why will create blocks that stop the manifestation process. Trust that you have put your intentions out there and made it known. The rest is out of your hands to an extent; granted there may be actions required for you to take in order to fulfill the desires of your destiny. They will come to you in divine timing. Listen to your intuition.

By focusing on abundance, you will draw more abundance into your life. If you are coming from a place of fear and lack, unfortunately, then those are the things that will follow. Like other methodologies mentioned in this book, it can take some practice to get your mind to be trained on a positive outlook. Once you get into a habit of having the higher vibrational frequency of positive dreams and desires you hold within, it will become like second nature. Sure, there will still be times where something isn't exactly going according to plan and you may want to dip into a low vibe feeling like sadness or fear, but you should be able to keep that in perspective if you are in a habit of being typically higher vibe.

# CHAPTER 9 RECAP: THINGS TO PONDER AND PRACTICE

1. Don't let little hang-ups get you down, stay focused on positivity.
2. Start a journal or note pad of your thoughts, intentions, and dreams.
3. Practice scripting by writing your dreams as if they have happened already.
4. Be grateful for everything you have.
5. What you think about is drawn to your life through the law of attraction.
6. Don't dwell on the outcome. Instead, wish and release.

# CHAPTER 10 – SELF CARE & FINAL THOUGHTS

One could argue that this entire book is essentially a guide on many different actions of self-care; however, I wanted to dedicate a specific chapter on this as it is all too often overlooked. Taking care of your mind, body, and spirit is not only important at maintaining health but in prevention of stress-related illnesses. You are in control of your thoughts, and thoughts become things. If you can work on controlling your thoughts on being positive, your life will benefit as a result. Have you ever looked at someone who is a pessimist and seen that their own negative outlook is putting a damper on their health? Is that person their own worst enemy?

Often it is easier to be on the outside looking in, but this is a good reminder for you to be conscious of yourself and your own needs. Make time for the things that make you feel good and smile! Getting your hair done, getting a massage, manicure, or just making the time to do a workout at home all counts as self-care. Setting a time to meditate as mentioned previously in this book is extremely helpful in gaining focus, patience, and for working on various chakras as well as mindfulness.

Get out and move around! Everything is energy, using energy in a positive way will cause more positivity to come to you. Take in some fresh air and enjoy nature whenever possible. If the availability of doing things like getting an appointment with a spa or self-care isn't available, try doing things yourself that make you feel good!

Some of my favorites to get an at-home spa experience is to light some candles or diffuse some essential oils and soak my feet in Epsom salt. I will often have a cup of tea while doing this as well as putting on a face mask or eye mask. Such a great, refreshing feeling! You are the artist of your own beautiful surroundings so make the most of what you can!

Use your intuition to guide you and have fun with it! Smile! Don't be your own worst enemy; be your own best friend! You are reading this for a reason and meant to see this message; nothing is by chance and it is all a part of a larger picture. Trust that the universe has your back and things will pan out as they are supposed to. You are amazing! Thank you for being here!

# ABOUT THE AUTHOR

A lifelong learner, Elliot has been on a journey of wellness research for years. He has acquired vast knowledge through completing courses, obtaining certifications, reading books, and participating in live and online events.

He is excited to be able to share from a fountain of amazing sources what he has learned, tried, and tested from the teachings.

As part of sharing the wealth of knowledge, he recently co-developed the website www.oneboolane.com with his soulmate Joe as a resource blog for inspiring others. As a thank you for reading this book, you can receive a free feng shui bagua worksheet via email (PDF).

To keep up-to-date with other book developments, and for your free gift, sign up for email updates through www.oneboolane.com and click contact. Subject line FREEGIFT.

Visit @oneboolane on Instagram for additional content, pictures, and stories. Enjoy the journey.

# APPENDIX

**Heather Askinosie** – Co-author of <u>Crystal Muse,</u> author of <u>Crystal 365</u>, cofounder of www.energymuse.com

**Craig Beck** – Author of <u>The Switch</u>, <u>Millionaire Mind</u> www.craigbeck.com

**Gabrielle Bernstein** - Author or <u>Super Attractor</u>, <u>You are the Guru</u>, <u>You are Here</u>, and others www.gabbybernstein.com

**Rhonda Byrne** – Author of <u>The Secret</u>, <u>The Power</u>, and others www.thesecret.tv

**Kyle Gray** - Author of <u>Raise your Vibration</u>, and others www.kylegray.co.uk

**Neville Goddard** – Author of <u>Feeling is the Secret</u>, <u>Believe in it</u>, and others

**Esther Hicks and Jerry Hicks** - The Law of Attraction, and others www.abraham-hicks.com

**Napolean Hill** – Author of <u>Think and Grow Rich</u>, <u>Master Key</u>, and others www.naphill.org

**Laura Lynne Jackson** - Author of <u>Signs: The Secret Language of the Universe</u>, and others www.lauralynnejackson.com

**Sarah Prout** - Author of <u>Dear Universe</u>, www.sarahprout.com

**James Van Praagh** - Author and course instructor *Healer, Psychic, Medium* www.vanpraagh.com